KETOGENIC DIET

COMPLETE GUIDE TO KETOGENIC DIET MADE EASY FOR WEIGHT LOSS AND HEALTHY LIFE

BY
J. MACHUCA

I0440190

TABLE OF CONTENTS

INTRODUCTION

CHAPTER 1: OVERVIEW ON THE KETOGENIC DIET:
EATING FATS WITHOUT GAINING FAT!
SOURCES OF ENERGY FOR YOUR BODY
WHAT ABOUT KETONES
HOW BODY ADJUSTS TO KETOGENIC DIET
HOW TO REACH KETOSIS
ADVANTAGES OF KETOGENIC OVER OTHER DIETS

CHAPTER 2: ESSENTIAL FACTS TO LEARN BEFORE HITTING
ON THE KETOGENIC DIET
3 TYPES OF KETOGENIC DIETS
SEEKING PROFESSIONAL ADVICE

CHAPTER 3: THE BENEFITS OF DROPPING THE CARBS
BURNS FATS FAST!
KETONES ARE HARMLESS AND EASY TO DISPOSE
KETOSIS HANDLES YOUR SWEET TOOTH
CONTROLS INSULIN LEVEL
MAKES YOU FEEL LESS HUNGRY

CHAPTER 4: GETTING STARTED WITH THE KETOGENIC
DIET
A GUIDE TO PROTEIN, CARB AND FAT INTAKE
PROTEIN
CARBOHYDRATES
FATS

CHAPTER 5: MYTHS AND MISCONCEPTIONS
COMMON MYTHS AND MISCONCEPTIONS

CHAPTER 6: HEALTHY TIPS AND FAT BURNING RECIPES
FOR A HEALTHY DIET
HEALTHY TIPS FOR MAXIMIZING SUCCESS ON KETOGENIC DIET
BONUS!
CONCLUSION

INTRODUCTION

If you are looking for some solution to your weight problem, you might as well consider the Ketogenic diet. Although this diet approach to healthy eating is quite confusing, it's amazing and challenging to know that you can burn fats by actually consuming more fats. This really sounds ironic! However, many studies have back up this diet approach and had been proven by many to be effective.

Through this book, "Getting Easy with the Ketogenic Diet: A Practical Guide to Ketogenic Dieting Made Easy for Weight Loss and Healthier Life", you will be introduced to a kind of diet that has gained global popularity and is still trending even after years since its discovery.

It is the aim of this book, to introduce the Ketogenic diet and show you how it is beneficial to people who need to lose weight or maintain their ideal body built through a healthy lifestyle. This book will provide you with a step-by-step procedure on Ketogenic diet including its precautionary measures. Lastly, also included in this book are delectable recipes on low-carb and high-fat dishes which are essential ingredients of a Ketogenic diet plus healthy tips to maximize your potentials of success in the ketogenic diet...

OVERVIEW ON THE KETOGENIC DIET: EATING FATS WITHOUT GAINING FAT!

If you want to lose fat, avoid taking fats!

This had been the common notions in the past and even leading health research institutes strongly backed this up. However, many scientific studies have come out to prove this wrong! These scientific studies reveal that if we want to lose fat faster, we must increase our fat intake BUT limit our consumption of carbohydrates.

The ketogenic diet was first recognized in 1920's as a way of controlling epilepsy in children, but in recent years, this principle was adopted in the development of a highly effective diet plan geared towards losing weight fast.

Recognized as an efficient high in fat and low in carbohydrates kind of diet, the Ketogenic diet is designed to provide an adequate number of calories and protein for gaining a healthy weight. The primary objective of the Ketogenic diet is to prompt the body to burn fat instead of carbohydrates, which can result in a quick loss of weight.

When high fat content causes concern in a health-conscious society which would normally associate 'fat' with 'bad', it is surprising to know that there is a good kind of fat. Good fats are healthy and are a necessary part of a controlled and balanced diet.

On the other hand, carbohydrates can cause a spike in blood sugar levels which eventually leads to obesity and signifies low energy levels. Part of the appeal of the Ketogenic diet is its ability to achieve fast weight loss and is, therefore, ideal to those who had managed to accumulate so many fats.

This diet eliminates intake of foods high in carbohydrates such as starchy fruits and veggies, sugar, pasta, and bread while increasing your fat content. A typical meal consists of chicken or fish with green vegetables and finally closes with a typical dessert of fruits filled generously with cream. Breakfast can be bacon and eggs while a cheese-filled snack accompanied by cucumber is an excellent way of filling up your day.

There are just too many variants of the Ketogenic diet and some include a more relaxed version of the regime. The first few days of the diet involves the body adapting to several ways of eating which can cause you to feel 'withdrawn'. This is likely to happen since most of our common meal consists of food heavy in starch and sugar.

While undergoing this transition period, those who are into the ketogenic diet will begin to experience an increase in energy levels in addition to fast weight loss. Enjoying your meal is essential if the diet is to prove to be sustainable, hence, this diet can be very enjoyable. You can fill your meal with delicious fish, steaks, eggs, bacon, and fruits with heavy cream.

Low level of complex carbohydrates will be reintroduced once excess weight has been trimmed down for long term weight maintenance.

Sources of Energy for your Body

Your body needs energy in all its activities. Primarily, it sources energy from carbohydrates, fats, and even from proteins. If you limit your carbohydrate intake to 30 grams or less, your body is forced to search for other alternative sources to fuel it. This other source is from fat and your body can also manufacture carbohydrates from protein and glycerol, one of the fat's components.

What About Ketones

With the exception of the brain and nervous system, every organ in your body can use fatty acids as an alternative energy source. In fact, the brain and the nervous system can function effectively even without glucose or carbohydrates because they can source up to 75 percent of their energy from ketones. Ketones are produced by an incomplete breakdown of fatty acids in the liver. These ketones are the primary sources of fuel for the brain and nervous system.

If you are adopting the Ketogenic diet, the body starts manufacturing more ketones and greatly reduces the use of glucose. Simultaneously, the conversion of protein to energy is likewise reduced and this is very important when you are trying to keep a lean body mass or muscles. The more muscles you generate, the more calories your body is likely to burn. This process is what makes ketogenic diet so effective.

How Body Adjusts to Ketogenic Diet

The body needs approximately three weeks to completely adjust to the usage of fatty acids and ketones as an energy source. Hence, on your first few days on a ketogenic diet is likely to be difficult. You will find it hard to focus and you will feel so weak and will even experience some nausea. Your body had been used to carbohydrates for so long that once you lower your carbohydrate level, your body is sure to experience a big shock! Only when your body starts to adjust will you then start to benefit from the ketogenic diet.

As you start eating high fat and low carbohydrates diet, you will be strongly influencing two important hormones in your body – insulin and glucagon. Insulin transports nutrients from the blood to cells like when glucose is being transported to your muscles.

On the other hand, glucagon works in the opposite. It influences the cells to release the stored nutrients to the bloodstream. When there is a shortage of glucose, it encourages the liver to outsource glucose and then released into the blood where they are being transported to other cells of the body.

Once you lower the carbohydrate intake, the body will gradually start releasing less and less of insulin and more of glucagon. That will send the body to release fatty acids from the fat deposits and transport them to the liver where they are being metabolized. That leads to an increase in ketone production, bringing the body to a state called 'ketosis'.

How to Reach Ketosis

There are many different ketogenic diets and all are based on the principle that you lower the level of carbohydrate intake significantly. The ceiling level for the carbohydrate intake is 30-50 grams. However, this is the case to case depending on the individual. When you take less, then the faster you will reach your ketosis.

In a ketogenic diet, you also have to increase your fat intake as fat should represent the main source of calories in your diet. You should also take about 1-2 protein per kg or 1 gram of protein per pound so you will not lose lean body mass.

Advantages of Ketogenic Over Other Diets

- Ketones can suppress your appetite making it an ideal one as you won't be craving for   more food while on this diet.
- Minimal muscle loss though you will experience some loss of strength especially at the start of a program diet.
- Ketones help improve moods.
- You can enjoy your meal without facing or worrying over its ill-effects afterward.

2

ESSENTIAL FACTS TO LEARN BEFORE HITTING ON THE KETOGENIC DIET

Once you consider losing weight through the ketogenic diet, you must also be aware of some important information before actually hitting on the diet.

The ketogenic diet was first used in the treatment of seizure attacks on epileptic children. Now, the diet was popular among dieters who are passionate on losing weight quickly without compromising their pleasure in eating. Though there are some risks, these are easily eliminated through adequate knowledge on the subject and by following the rules. Especially for beginners, they need to strictly adhere to every rule. They need to have some overview of the diet before deciding to take a leap on it.

For those with health problems, it is crucial to seek advice from your health care provider so he can assist you in this diet plan and likewise monitor your condition to make sure that the ketogenic diet will not have an ill effect on the patient.

3 Types of Ketogenic Diets

The ketogenic diet is a high-fat low carbohydrate diet with adequate protein thrown in the meal. It is further divided into three types and depending on one's daily calorie needs, the percentage differs. Diets are often prepared on a ratio level such as 4:1 or 2:1 with the first number indicating the total fat amount in the diet compared to the protein and carbohydrate combined in each meal.

Standard - SKD

The first diet is the Standard or the SKD and is designed for individuals who are not active or lead a sedentary lifestyle. The meal plan limits the dieter to eat a net of 20-50 grams of carbohydrates. Fruits or vegetables that are starchy are restricted from the diet. In order for the diet to be effective, one must strictly follow the meal plan. Butter, vegetable oil, and heavy creams are used heavily to replace carbohydrates in the diet.

Targeted – TKD

The targeted is too lax in comparison to the standard (SKD) diet as it allows you to consume carbohydrates in regulated portions so it will not create an impact on the ketosis. TKD also helps the one in diet have some regular exercise.

Cyclical – CKD

This level is preferable for those who are too active with their physical workout and not recommended for beginners. This diet requires the dieter to stick to an SKD plan for five days in a week and the loading up on carbs for the next two days. It is important that everyone who is using the ketogenic diet must stick to a strict compliance of the diet regiment to be successful.

Seeking Professional Advice

It is essential that before you decide to go on this diet, you should go and check with your physician if you have any special concern about it. It is hazardous to start with a ketogenic plan if you have any pre-existing health condition especially those that involve kidney or heart problem. Be sure that the following health issues are properly ruled out before going on a ketogenic diet.

Consult your physician about implementing a Ketogenic diet if you have any of these conditions:

- Gall bladder disease (Active)
- History of pancreatitis
- Liver Dysfunction
- Poor nutritional status
- Fat Digestion Failure
- History of kidney failure
- Bypass surgery for gastric ailment
- Abdominal cyst and tumors
- Pregnancy and lactation
- Decreased gastrointestinal motility

There are some medical practitioners who got little training on nutrition and don't have enough understanding of the general effect of foods on the body. Some are even oriented that ketosis is dangerous and hence, they have little knowledge about ketogenic diets. Physicians with this kind of mentality are likely to push you back.

Further, there are some physicians who get nutritional ketosis confused with a dangerous condition called ketoacidosis, but these are two entirely different conditions. Ketoacidosis is one of the many concerns for Type 1 Diabetes and for those whose bodies are unable to properly process insulin.

Ketoacidosis is usually developed when a person with type 1 diabetes develops a serious health condition like infection, heart attack or other debilitating illness. It is usually accompanied by high level of sugar in the blood, dehydration and is precipitated by the person's inability to administer proper amount of injected insulin.

3

THE BENEFITS OF DROPPING THE CARBS

T

he ketogenic diet is now one of the hottest approaches to weight loss as more people are embracing the idea of an extremely low carb diet, which aims to be in a state of ketosis. Ketosis as simply described is the state of the body where it is burning fat as fuel as opposed to glucose. One may be able to achieve this state, largely by depriving the body of glucose through a certain dietary plan. Here are some benefits you can derive from ketogenic diets.

Burns Fats Fast!

Being in a ketosis state allows the body to process fat quickly and use it as fuel in a way that no other state or condition allows as easily. Carbohydrates are much easier to convert into energy, hence, when you are providing plenty of these to your body, you need to burn and use all before your body will start converting and using fat for fuel.

Ketones are Harmless and Easy to Dispose

Any ketones that are in excess can't harm your body system in any way. Any ketones produce and which are not needed by your body are simply released through urine. You can always check every morning if you are in a state of ketosis by checking on your urine through the use of urine testing strips.

Ketosis Handles your Sweet Tooth

As your body gets used to being in the state of ketosis, it will no longer crave for sugar but will, in fact, prefer protein as a fuel source in oppose to sugar. So for people who normally have a "sweet tooth", your system will actually prefer ketones over glucose so don't be surprised if you find yourself no longer attracted to sweets and desserts!

Controls Insulin Level

Another benefit of being in a ketogenic state is its ability to control your insulin level. Insulin's primary purpose is to break down carbohydrates and converting them into glucose. It is also responsible for your cravings for sweet and starchy foods. Controlling it to a healthy level is one of the objectives of weight loss.

Makes you Feel Less Hungry

Lastly, being healthy is not based on the quantity of food that you eat, but rather on the quality of what you are consuming. Most people got into the habit of eating too much leading to obesity which is one of risk factors for many deadly medical conditions.

The majority of the people who are into ketogenic diet report that the diet makes them significantly less hungry than when they are into a non-ketogenic state. It is typical for a person to stick to a diet or just any diet when you are not fighting against great cravings and hunger while you're on it. A person tends to lose his control and self-discipline to appease his hunger once it arises. So, not having to deal with them makes it indeed easier for you to finish what you had started with your dieting plan.

Now that you are sufficiently oriented on the benefits of being in a state of ketosis, it's probably easier for you to decide if you want to give the ketogenic diet a try?

4

T

o get started with the Ketogenic diet, there are 3 steps to a customized Ketogenic Diet.

- Know your ideal body weight.
  To get your ideal body weight, you can use some online calculators like the one here: http://www.calculator.net/ideal-weight-calculator.html.
- Establish a daily requirement of calorie to maintain ideal body weight.
- Determine the quantity of protein, carb and fat to take based on ideal weight and calories.

A Guide to Protein, Carb and Fat Intake

Protein

On average, the ratio of your protein intake to your lean body mass or ideal body is 1-1.5 g: 1kg.

For instance, you weigh 150 lbs. and have a lean body mass of 100 lbs. In order to take the average optimum amount of your protein intake, begin your calculation at 1g/kg/LBM and also take the higher end using 1.5g/kg/LBM. Now, since you have your weigh scale set by pounds, don't forget to divide it by 2.2 to convert it into kilograms.

Taken step-by-step:

1. 100 lbs. LBM / 2.2 = 45 kg. LBM
2. 45 x 1g = 45g of protein (lower end range)
3. 45 x 1.5g =67.5g of protein (higher end range)

Therefore, your average optimum intake of protein should be somewhere between 45-68g daily.

Carbohydrates

Essentially, when it comes to handling carb daily is not to exceed at 60g. However, this may vary from case-to-case. If you have severe problems in insulin, metabolism or is diabetic, you need to be very strict on your carbohydrates.

On the other hand, if you have a great amount of lean body mass in your body or do exercise a lot, then you may need to take more of it in order to stay in ketosis. This speaks true to those who do vigorous exercises like cycling and those who are into sport.

Now, if you want to lose weight, you need to adjust your carbohydrates to below 30 grams daily. Another tip you can use if limiting your carb doesn't work out—use the lower end of your average protein intake.

Fats

Calories from fats make up the balance of your calories after taking out the carb and protein calories. We have included two examples that you can observe.

Sample #1: Person A is overweight. She would like to go down to an ideal weight of 150 lbs. In order to achieve her objective, she was advised to take 1800 calories daily, taking 1kg per kg of her LBM for protein and only 30g of carbohydrates.

Calculation:

1. Calculate the protein: 150/2.2 = 68 x 1g = 68g or 272 calories
2. Calculate the carb: 30g = 120 calories
3. Combine calories from protein and carbohydrates: 272 + 120 = 392
4. Calculate the fats: That is 1800 (from total calories) – 392 (total from carb and protein calories) = 1,408 fat calories.
5. To convert fats into grams: 1408/ 9= 156g of fat daily

Sample #2: Person B's ideal weight is 185 lbs. To limit her calories into 2500 per day with 60g of carbohydrates to calculate at the higher end 1.5g since she exercises for an hour daily.

Calculation:

1. Calculate the protein: 185/ 2.2 = 84 x 1.5g = 124g or 504 calories
2. Calculate the carb: 60g = 240 calories
3. Combine calories from protein and carbohydrates: 504 + 240= 744 calories
4. Calculate fats: 2500 (from total calories) – 744 (total from carb and protein calories) = 1,756 fat calories
5. To convert fat grams into calories: 1,756/ 9= 195g of fat daily

Important Rules in Observing Ketogenic Diet

For best results, here are some important rules and guidelines you have to observe.

Rule #1: Eat only the foods listed herein

If you want to take other foods, you must—first and foremost—check the serving size. Take note of the amount of carbohydrates as well. Remember that you should have 5g or less per serving for vegetables; and 2g or less per serving for meat and dairy.

Rule #2: Eat only the following foods when you're hungry

And always bear in mind to *never* overeat. Additionally, foods rich in protein may be grilled, microwaved, boiled, baked, stir-fried, roasted, sautéed and fried in their natural fats (do not add breading, flour, or cornmeal).

Seafood, poultry and meat (fresh or frozen, but be mindful of additives for the frozen stuff)

- **Important**: Keep away from whey protein at least until you achieve your goals for weight loss. It actually increases the potency of insulin.
- **Seafood and/or fish**: (prefer the wild-caught ones) tuna, trout, bass, anchovies, salmon, sardines, cod, flounder, calamari, catfish, mackerel, herring, snapper, scrod, halibut, and sole.
- **Shellfish**: lobsters, crabs (with the exception of processed crab meat since it sugar and lots of additives), scallops, squid, mussels, oysters and shrimps.
- **Canned**: Tuna and salmon but always check the label first. (Never with the breaded and fried seafood.)
- **Poultry**: chicken, Cornish hen, turkey, duck, goose, quail and/or any kind of poultry.
- **Whole eggs**: Can be prepared in different ways— hard-boiled, soft-boiled, deviled, omelet, scrambled, poached and fried.
- **Meat**: (preferably from those that eat grass) beef, goat, goat, lamb, veal or wild game

- **Pork**: pork chops, pork loin, Boston butt and ham (but watch out for added sugars).
- **Bacon and sausage**: Watch out for carb which should only 2g or less.
- **Soy products**: tofu, edamame and tempeh (but they could be high source of carbohydrates so be conscious about that).

Rule #3: Eat one cup of fiber-rich vegetables and 1-2 cups of greens every day for your Vitamin K intake

- **Salad greens**: all varieties of cabbage and lettuce, all varieties of greens including mustard, beet, turnip and collard, spinach, parsley, kale, chives, and chard.
- **Fiber-rich veggies**: Broccoli, cauliflower, radishes, bean sprouts, wax beans, green or string beans, asparagus, bell pepper, Brussels sprouts, carrot (raw), cucumber, mushrooms, celery, rhubarb, water chestnuts, turnip, tomatoes (raw), snow peas, summer squash, zucchini, bok choy, bamboo shoots, jicama, and okra. (Tomatoes and carrots are high in sugar; hence, they should be eaten raw and should be limited to half cup serving only.

Rule #4: Use only the fats listed here

Take note that saturated animal fats are given more importance compared to those extracted from vegetable oils (e.g. canola, corn, sunflower, grapeseed, and safflower). Refrain from taking in polyunsaturated fatty acids as they cause inflammation to our bodies.

For cooking or heating process

- **Organic**: coconut oil, coconut cream concentrate, coconut butter, olive oil (cold-pressed), lard (not hydrogenated), duck fat, chicken fat, butter (for low-temperature frying) and red palm oil (taken only in small amounts)
- Ghee butter

For cold dressings

- Mayonnaise: if you can do homemade mayo using avocado and macadamia oils, they're much preferable.
- Seed oils and most nut oils (do not undergo heating process and limit usage): almond oil, flaxseed oil and sesame oil.
- Macadamia oil
- Avocado oil

Rule #5: Limit your intake with these foods

- **Veggies rich in fats**
  - Avocado: half of it daily
  - Olives (green or black variants): up to 7 daily
- **Cheese** (up to 4 oz. daily)
  - Block or whipped cream cheese, no added whey
  - Cheddar and Swiss (any hard and old cheese)
  - Mozzarella, Brie, Camembert, blue and goat cheeses (soft cheeses)
  - Important: Avoid the processed kinds. Also, the carb count should be 1g per serving.

- **Mayonnaise** (up to 4 tbsp. daily)
  - Low-carb kind like the Hellman's and the Duke's.
  - Important: Observe less than 1g carb per serving.
- **Dairy Cream** (up to 4 tbsp. daily)
  - Sour, heavy and whipping creams
  - Important: Check the label and avoid those with whey. Stay away from milk and half-n-half since they contain too many carbohydrates.
- **Snacks**
  - Nuts and nut flours (less than 1 oz. daily)
  - Pork rinds (not exceeding 2 servings daily)
  - Important: Do not eat snacks with or made of whey protein.
- **Condiments**
  - Pickles: (be sure to check on labels for serving size) Choose sugar and dill-free kinds observing no more than 2 servings daily.
  - Salad dressing: It's best to make your very own dressing using oil and non- balsamic vinegar; or the mixture of sour cream and spicing, to thin out using water or cream.
  - Lemon or lime juice: up to 4 teaspoons daily
  - Ketchup: choose the low-sugar kind and take only 1 tablespoon daily.
  - Soy sauce: check labels for carb count and limit for up to 4 tablespoons daily.
  - Important: Stevia (or other artificial sweeteners) and spices should be taken only in small quantities.
- **Drinks and beverages**
  - Water
  - Decaffeinated coffee
  - Bouillon or clear broth
  - Unsweetened drinks: almond milk (2 cups daily), decaffeinated tea, herbal tea and flavored seltzer water

- **Other Snacks**
  - Feta cheese-stuffed olives
  - Raw or roasted nuts
  - Sugar-free, cured beef jerky
  - Deviled or hard-boiled eggs with mayonnaise or sour cream spread
  - Bacon, tomato chunks with cream cheese or mayo in lettuce leaf
  - Mayo, cream cheese and tuna mix set on round cuts of cucumber
  - Butter-fried macadamia nuts with a dash of cinnamon
  - Pecans with thinly sliced blue cheese
  - Boiled or steamed shrimp with dill mayonnaise
  - Greek yogurt enhanced with ginger, cinnamon, cardamom and sweetener
  - Pepperoni slices with string cheese

5

T

he key to a happy life is to have a healthy body and for you to have a healthy body, you need to live a healthy lifestyle. A healthy lifestyle is always linked to a well-balanced diet, regular exercise, and sufficient quality sleep.

Relative to this, there are different types of diets that claim to embody a healthy lifestyle. A low-carb diet signifies a low-carb lifestyle as it evolves through a diet, which restricts the consumption of carbohydrates-rich foods such as those, found in starchy fruits and vegetables (root crops), and grains. Instead of these foods, they are replaced by protein-rich foods like fish, lean meat, milk, poultry, and fats – butter, vegetable oil, etc.

The thrust of a low-carb diet and lifestyle is towards losing weight but it can lead to other health benefits beyond weight loss including the reduction of risk factors associated with diabetes, heart disease, and metabolic syndrome.

Common Myths and Misconceptions

There are a number of misconceptions and myths associated with ketogenic diets, a primary low-carb diet. Many are led to believe that these carbohydrates-controlled diets prohibit eating of fruits, vegetables, and alcohol. Other misconceptions focus as well on the diet's side effects such as increasing cholesterol levels, causing kidney malfunction and promoting heart disease.

Here are some of the few common misconceptions and wrong connotations about the ketogenic diet.

Myth: Both Low-Carb and High-Fat Diets Increase Cholesterol Levels

Fact: There are many testimonials scattering across the internet testifying to the fact that those who follow the ketogenic diet have improvements in blood sugar and cholesterol level.

Myth: Low-carb Diets Promote Heart Disease

Fact: A number of studies prove that low-carb diets have higher chances of reducing the major markers for heart disease risks which include regulating high blood pressure, reducing glucose, triglycerides and inflammation while increasing good cholesterol level.

Myth: People on Low Carb Diets are Prohibited from Drinking Alcohol.

Fact: Most alcoholic beverages are low in carbohydrates though they have high calorie-content. A regular beer carries about 12 grams of carbohydrates per 12 ounces serving. The key here is moderate consumption.

Myth: Low-carb Diet can Cause Kidney or Liver Damage Due to High Protein

Fact: Studies show that carb-controlled ketogenic can heal the kidneys rather than put strains on them. This is due to the fact that the amount of protein and fat consumption recommended in low carb diets are not harmful to the kidneys and liver.

Myth: Low-carb Means Elimination of Fruits, Vegetables and Other Source of Carbohydrates

Fact: Low-carb diet specifically eliminates consumption of "starchy" fruits and vegetables or those that are high in carbohydrate contents. Not all fruits and vegetables have this "culprit" carbs. Fruits like watermelon, berries, and apricots can be eaten in moderate amount.

Myth: Low-carb Diets are not Suitable for Long Term and Weight Maintenance

Fact: It is always possible to be a lifetime low-carb dieter to maintain weight. In fact, most ketogenic dieters had adopted this as a healthy lifestyle.

Myth: Low-carb Diets Causes Mass Degeneration and Total Body Water Instead of Fat Loss

Fact: Studies reveal that low-carb lifestyle favorably affects the physical composition of the body. People on low-carb diet are losing more body fats and less lean body mass or muscles compared to those who were into a low-fat diet.

Myth: Glucose in the Carbohydrate Form is the Sole Source of Energy for the Brain

Fact: While brain cells need some glucose to function, they are likewise flexible and can utilize fuel from ketones and fatty acids which are important fuels for many cell types in the body.

Myth: A Low-carb Diet Causes Insufficiency in Vitamins and Minerals.

Fact: Ketogenic Diet allows dieters to eat nutrient-filled foods including meat, eggs, fruits and vegetables. Adhering to a correct diet plan can avoid dietary deficiencies.

Myth: Ketogenic Diets are Dangerous, Low in Fiber and Hazardous to your Colon

Fact: Ketogenic studies is known for their neuroprotective effects and involvement in the therapy for medical conditions like Alzheimer's disease, some cancers, diabetes, Parkinson's illness, and epilepsy. Further, Ketogenic diets include more food rich in fibers such as cabbage, spinach, and salads and in fact, make up a significant portion of the carbohydrate calories allowed.

6

HEALTHY TIPS AND FAT BURNING RECIPES FOR A HEALTHY DIET

S
ince the peak of low-carb diets in the 90's, ketogenic diets are still very highly accepted as effective, weight loss maintenance diets. Most of those who are into this diet had in fact adopted it as a healthy lifestyle. Here are some tips for you on how to reach your maximum potential for success on the ketogenic diet.

Healthy Tips for Maximizing Success on Ketogenic Diet

Drink a lot of water

Your body will find hard time retaining water while you're on a ketogenic staying. Hence, it is important to stay hydrated all the time. Experts are recommending a minimum of 3 liters a day for men and 2.2 liters for women. While you aren't sure, what's the right amount for you, the color of your urine is a good sign of proper hydration. If it is clear and light yellow, then you are likely to be properly hydrated. So always make sure to keep a bottle of water handy.

Always Remember the Fat!

Don't forget that fat in a ketogenic diet is an essential element in the absence of sufficient carbohydrates. Just as we need to fuel our body to stay active and energetic, we need fats. Nonetheless, don't forget to choose the good kind of fats. Fill yourself up with healthy, unsaturated fats like avocados, nuts, olives, and seed.

Curb your Carbs!

Each individual has different calorie level requirement. White some need to stick to a strict low-carb diet that requires them to consume less than 20g of carb daily, others find it comfortable to stay in ketosis while consuming 50-100g of carbs per day. The only way to know this is through trial and error and this may take some time. Using a urinalysis strips for ketones will also help you find out your carbohydrates limit.

Be patient

Though ketogenic diet is said to be a fast fat burning activity, remember that each individual is different and effects of ketogenic on a person may vary based on various factors. So don't expect to lose your weight in a day or two and don't freak out when the scale doesn't show any sign of weight loss or just a slight weight change for a number of days. You can also use some other metrics like your body measurements to see changes beyond what the scale shows.

BONUS!!!!

T

  o finally water your mouth with delectable dishes even while you're on a diet, here's your bonus for reading this book. Here are 3 mouth-watering dishes that will surely spice up your diet.

These low-carb and delectable food dishes are just perfect for pampering your taste buds even while on a ketogenic diet. From here, you can always work on a variety of ways to create your own recipes out of this selection to come out with new exciting and scrumptious variations

BAKED BACON AND EGG

Ingredients

- Butter (2 tablespoon)
- Large eggs (4 pieces)
- Cheddar cheese, grated (1 cup)
- Heavy cream, heated to lukewarm (1 cup)
- Cooked bacon, crumbled (8 slices)
- Salt and pepper to taste

Directions

1. Heat the oven to 350°F. Butter 4 small glass or ceramic bowls (about 6 0z.).
2. Break an egg on each bowl. Individually top each egg with ¼ cup of cheese and ¼ cup of heated cream.
3. Season with salt and pepper to taste.
4. Bake for 15 minutes or until the cheese if fully melted and the egg whites have turned white.
5. Top each egg with two slices of bacon and serve immediately.

Blueberry Lemon Muffins

Ingredients

- Almond Flour (2 cups)
- Heavy cream (1 cup)
- Eggs (2 large)
- Melted butter (1/8 cup)
- Artificial Sweetener (5 packets)
- Baking soda (1/2 tsp.)
- Lemon extract or flavoring (1/2 tsp.)
- Dried lemon zest (1/2 tsp.)
- Salt (1/4 tsp.)
- Fresh blueberries (4 oz.)

Directions

1. Preheat oven while placing cupcake papers in muffin molds.
2. Combine almond flour and cream. Add one egg at a time and stir until the mixture is well mixed.
3. Add butter, spices, sweetener, baking soda and flavoring and blend. Also add the blueberries and mix until evenly distributed.
4. Spoon mixture into each hole of the muffin molds about half-full.
5. Bake until golden brown and let it cool for a few minutes before serving.

CHOCOLATE STRAWBERRY PROTEIN DRINK

Ingredients

- Unsweetened almond milk (16 oz.)
- Heavy cream (4 0z.)
- Jay Robb Chocolate Whey Isolate powder (2 scoops)
- DaVinci Sugar Free Strawberry Syrup (1 tbsp.)
- *Optional*: Crushed ice

Directions

Put all ingredients in a blender and blend until smooth in consistency.

R

eaching this far end of your reading had somehow enlightened you on the facts about ketogenic diet and had probably ironed out any doubts, which have been probably troubling you before.

While you have decided to embrace the ketogenic diet approach, you will not only be dealing with physical discipline but with mental and emotional perseverance and control as well. Embracing the Ketogenic Diet, as a lifestyle will not only improve your physical built but will eventually provide you a healthy well being and a happier life ahead.

As you keep on watching your ideal weight while you are on this diet, may you share to others your experience as well. Sharing to others this book is a great way of promoting a healthy lifestyle and reducing health risks. The best way to a peaceful place to live in is through having healthy and happy people surrounding you. Give your best shot through this diet and acquire a stronger and a healthier you!

www.ingramcontent.com/pod-product-compliance
Lightning Source LLC
Chambersburg PA
CBHW050848290526
45792CB00002B/570